DHEA: Your Fount

Copyright © 2015 by Susan l

All rights reserved. No part of this book may be reproduced or transmitted in any form or by any means, electronic or mechanical, including photocopying, recording, or by any information storage or retrieval system, without permission in writing from the Publisher.

Dr. Susan's Healthy Living
drsusanshealthyliving.com

Facebook.com/DrSusanRichards
drsusanshealthyliving@gmail.com
(650) 561-9978

Mention of specific companies or products in this book does not suggest endorsement by the author or publisher. Internet addresses and telephone numbers for resources provided in this book were accurate at the time it went to press.

ISBN 978-1511977432

Note

The information in this book is meant to complement the advice and guidance of your physician, not replace it. It is very important that any person who has medical problems be evaluated by a physician. If you are under the care of a physician, you should discuss any major changes in your regimen with him or her. Because this is a book and not a medical consultation, keep in mind that the information presented here may not apply in your particular case. In view of individual medical requirements, new research, and government regulations, it is the responsibility of the reader to validate health practices and treatments with a physician or health service.

Table of Contents

Chapter 1: Understanding DHEA 5
    Benefits of DHEA 7

Chapter 2: The Chemistry of DHEA 8
    DHEA's Role in Your Body 10
    How DHEA Deficiency Occurs 10
    How Diet, Health and Lifestyle Affect DHEA Levels ... 11
    Looking Ahead 14

Chapter 3: DHEA and Peak Performance 15
    Physical Vitality and Energy 15
    Determination and Perseverance in Pursuing Goals ... 17
    The Ability to Remain Calm Under Pressure 19
    Optimism and Vision 21

Chapter 4: DHEA and Your Health 23
    Menopausal Symptoms 23
    Balance Thyroid Levels 24
    Stress and Anxiety 25
    Depression 25
    Insomnia 26
    Loss of Libido 26
    Poor Memory and Mental Fog 27
    Osteoporosis 29
    Cardiovascular Disease 31
    Excess Weight 33
    Diabetes 34
    Weakened Immune Function 35
    Asthma 38
    Cancer 39

Chapter 5: Testing for DHEA Deficiency 41
    Testing for DHEA Deficiency 42
    Ranges of DHEA Levels 43

Chapter 6: Support Your Own Production of DHEA 44
    Boost Your Adrenal Function 45

Chapter 7: Bioidentical DHEA 71
    Using DHEA 71
    Supplementing With DHEA 73
    A Caution on Taking DHEA 75
    Summary 78

About Susan Richards, M.D. 79
Notes 80
Notes 82

1

Understanding DHEA

DHEA is one of the most exciting sex hormones for women with benefits that affect almost every aspect of our health. Yet, for decades, the medical field believed that even though the body produced large amounts of this hormone, it seemed to have no apparent purpose.

As subsequent research studies on DHEA began to receive attention, both in the medical literature and in the popular press, it became apparent that this hormone actually has great importance in maintaining many aspects of our well-being. The benefits of this hormone are so wide-reaching that it is now recognized as one of our most important markers of aging.

Supplementing with DHEA is gaining more popularity among alternative health care practitioners as its benefits for easing menopausal symptoms and boosting heart and bone health have become increasingly apparent. Research studies suggest that it is a veritable "fountain of youth" when levels of DHEA are balanced and healthy in the body. I have seen the dramatic health benefits of DHEA therapy with my own patients, many of whom have felt better and been able to perform much more effectively in their lives with DHEA supplementation.

DHEA is the abbreviation for a long and complicated sounding hormone, dehydroepiandrosterone. It is known as a precursor hormone since it is one of the primary steroid sex hormones from which your body produces testosterone and estrogen. Although much of DHEA is converted into these other two hormones, some of it remains unchanged and it creates its own significant benefits within the body. Ninety percent of DHEA is produced by the adrenal glands, while some is also made in the ovaries, brain, and skin tissue.

I have written this book to share with you the amazing health and peak performance benefits of DHEA. I discuss how to evaluate your own DHEA levels and laboratory testing of DHEA. Most importantly, I share with you my program for how to increase the level of DHEA production within your own body through the use of powerful and effective nutritional supplements and herbs as well as valuable information on bioidentical DHEA therapy. In the following chart, I list many of its remarkable benefits.

Benefits of DHEA

Peak Performance Benefits

- Greater ability to cope with stressful events
- Elevated mood
- Feeling of well-being
- Decreased fat
- Lift in energy
- Leaner body
- Feeling relaxed
- Improved concentration
- Promotes deeper and more restorative sleep
- Increased muscle strength

Health Benefits

- Decreases the risk of heart disease
- Strengthens the immune system
- May be useful in the treatment of autoimmune diseases such as rheumatoid arthritis, lupus, ulcerative colitis, and multiple sclerosis
- May help prevent cancer
- Reduces body fat
- Lessens symptoms of menopause and osteoporosis in women
- May be useful in the treatment of diabetes, asthma, and burns
- Enhances mental clarity and acuity
- May enhance libido

2

The Chemistry of DHEA

In this chapter, we'll look at how DHEA is produced and its role within the body. We'll also examine why DHEA levels diminish and how we become deficient in this essential hormone.

Adrenal hormones such as DHEA are primarily produced from a substance called acetyl coenzyme A (acetyl CoA), as well as cholesterol. Acetyl CoA is a chemical produced in the liver, made from fatty acids and amino acids. It provides an important source of energy for the body as well as being a building block from which hormones are made. Cholesterol is a waxy, white, fatty material, widely distributed in all body cells. The cholesterol in the body is supplied by animal foods in the diet, such as eggs and organ meats. Your liver also produces a certain amount of cholesterol.

Once DHEA is produced by the adrenals, it travels through the bloodstream to cells throughout the body. Within the glands and sex organs, it is converted to testosterone and estrogen in both men and women. However, the conversion is predominantly to testosterone in males and to estrogen in females.

Certain DHEA is also converted in the liver to a sulfur compound when a molecule of sulfate (sulfur plus oxygen) is added to it. This new substance is referred to as DHEA-S. It is thought that DHEA is pre-dominantly produced in the morning. This form of the hormone is rapidly excreted through the kidneys.

In contrast, DHEA-S is eliminated slowly, so levels remain more constant in the body. Because of the two different rates of excretion, of the total amount of this hormone in the blood, about 90 percent is DHEA-S. Curiously, not all animals make DHEA in significant amounts. It is produced in abundance by just the primates, including humans, monkeys, apes, and gorillas.

Once DHEA is produced by the adrenals, it travels through the bloodstream to cells throughout the body. Within the glands and sex organs, it is converted to testosterone and estrogen. Some DHEA is also converted in the liver to a sulfur compound when a molecule of sulfate, which is sulfur plus oxygen, is added to it. This new substance is referred to as DHEA-S. It is thought that DHEA is pre-dominantly produced in the morning. This form of the hormone is rapidly excreted through the kidneys.

In contrast, DHEA-S is eliminated slowly, so levels remain more constant in the body. Because of the two different rates of excretion, of the total amount of this hormone in the blood, 90 percent is DHEA-S.

DHEA's Role in Your Body

DHEA travels through the bloodstream to cells throughout the body. It works at many levels in your body, supporting physical as well as mental and emotional well-being. DHEA has been shown to lessen the symptoms of menopause; increase stamina, improve mood, mental outlook, and your ability to handle stress; reduce body fat; and treat diabetes. It also enhances mental clarity and acuity, promotes confidence and assertiveness, and may even improve libido!

In addition, DHEA may help to decrease your risk of heart disease and cancer; promote healthy bones; strengthen your immune system; ease autoimmune diseases such as rheumatoid arthritis, systemic lupus erythematosus, and ulcerative colitis; and treat conditions as varied as multiple sclerosis, burns and asthma. This is quite a long and positive list of benefits that this awesome hormone provides! We will be exploring each of these benefits in greater detail later on in this book.

How DHEA Deficiency Occurs

Of all the steroid hormones in your body, DHEA is the most prevalent and circulates in the bloodstream in the highest concentrations. Women produce about

1-2 mg of DHEA-S per day. This production declines with age. A fetus has relatively high amounts of DHEA, which functions to ease the birth process. However, by the time an infant is six months old, DHEA production all but ceases, and only revives at age six to eight in preparation for puberty. Peak DHEA production is between the ages of 25 and 30; after this, production declines by as much as 10 percent per year. A person may feel the effects of this by their mid-40's. At age 80, you make only about 15 percent of what you produced in your 20's.

A study appearing in the Annals of the New York Academy of Sciences documents this. Sixty-four volunteers, between the ages of 20 and 40, had four times the levels of DHEA-S as 138 volunteers over age 85. Patients with major diseases such as atherosclerosis, cancer, and Alzheimer's also have significant deficiencies.

How Diet, Health and Lifestyle Affect DHEA Levels

In addition to the aging process, a poor diet, excessive stress, and lack of exercise can all lower DHEA levels.

Diet

Interestingly, eating an unhealthy diet of foods that in general stress our bodies, also affect our levels of DHEA. To maintain healthy levels of DHEA, it is best to eat a high nutrient content diet of whole foods. This includes lots of fresh vegetables and fruits, whole grains, legumes, raw seeds and nuts and organic, range-fed meats.

Avoid or reduce your intake of caffeinated beverages, products made with refined sugar and white flour, alcohol, excessive amounts of fruit juice, MSG, aspartame (NutraSweet), and foods to which you are allergic (wheat and dairy products are common offenders), since they all can stimulate the release of stress hormones, thereby reducing DHEA levels.

When various functions such as digestion and detoxification by the liver are impaired, or if you have elevated levels of HDL cholesterol, this can also have an impact on the production of precursor hormones such as DHEA.

Stress

Excessive levels of stress definitely reduce our production of DHEA. On the other hand, cultivating a peaceful and relaxed mood helps to increase our production. One study I found fascinating was done at the Institute of HeartMath in Boulder Creek, California. Researchers took DHEA samples from 28 volunteers, then asked them to listen to music specifically designed to promote a sense of peacefulness and emotional balance every day for one month. At the end of the month, researchers took a second DHEA sample from the volunteers. The results were impressive. Among all volunteers, levels of DHEA increased, on average 100 percent. For some, the levels tripled and even quadrupled. Since DHEA is a precursor hormone, this means that the hormones that arise from DHEA, such as testosterone and estrogen, are also more likely to increase with the use of the HeartMath program.

In addition to producing DHEA, your adrenal glands manufacture other hormones, including cortisol. Cortisol is released during times of extreme stress, be it physical, emotional, or mental. When you produce too much cortisol and not enough DHEA, you can throw your adrenal glands out of balance, and eventually strain them to the point of exhaustion. Because DHEA levels are already naturally decreasing as you get older, this imbalance can aggravate both perimenopausal and menopausal symptoms.

Exercise

A study highlighted in Age and Ageing showed that regular moderate aerobic exercise such as walking, swimming, or biking increased DHEA production in older people. This is another one of the many health benefits that regular exercise provides for women (and men) of all ages. Because of research such as this, I particularly recommend doing physical activeities at least 4 to 5 days a week in order to help restore your DHEA levels. Aim for 30 minutes to an hour per session, outdoors if possible.

Looking Ahead

A wealth of research on DHEA has begun mostly during the past few decades. These studies have examined many of the different physiological and psychological effects that DHEA produces within the body. In the next two chapters, we'll take a look at some of the more important ones.

3

DHEA and Peak Performance

A wealth of research on DHEA has begun to accumulate that is so positive that it makes DHEA seem like "a fountain of youth." These studies have reported increased energy, improved mood, better sleep quality, and a greater ability to remain calm and handle stress. I discuss many of these wonderful benefits of DHEA in this chapter.

Physical Vitality and Energy

DHEA supplementation helps increase physical energy and vitality in both women and men who are reaching mid-life and beyond when DHEA levels begin to diminish. This is of great benefit since fatigue is one of the most common complaints that I hear from patients.

In one research study, 17 women and 13 men between the ages of 40 to 70 years old were evaluated for the effects of DHEA on their well-being. The subjects were given 50 mg. of DHEA or a placebo every day for 3 months. 82percent of the women and 67 percent of the men taking DHEA noted an increase in their energy level and their sense of physical well-being.

They also enjoyed deeper, sounder sleep, an improved ability to deal with stress and a more balanced mood.

These results are not surprising, since DHEA is directly converted within the body into testosterone in men, and first testosterone and then estrogen in women.

Many of these positive traits of physical and emotional well-being are greatly diminished when women enter menopause and their levels of female hormones like DHEA-dependent estrogen and testosterone diminish.

DHEA even influences muscle mass and physical strength. This is more pronounced in men since DHEA directly converts into testosterone, the main male hormone. Testosterone is the hormone that directly influences muscle mass and strength. The more testosterone an individual has, the more likely he or she is to be well muscled. Teenage boys with high levels of DHEA and testosterone are more likely to have heavier beards, deeper voices, larger muscles, and even a higher sex drive than their less androgenized peers.

At the other end of the spectrum, my older male patients occasionally complain about a loss of muscle mass and muscle atrophy. These men have usually related these changes in their physical structure, often occurring with a decline in libido, to the aging process. Not surprisingly, these physical changes are often seen in their sixties and seventies, when DHEA as well as testosterone production normally declines in many men.

Loss of muscle mass, however, isn't just a male problem. Many of my female patients who are in the postmenopausal years complain about sagging and dropping of their breasts, buttocks and abdominal muscles that even regular fitness and workout routines don't seem to solve. DHEA can offer similar benefits to building muscular strength and tone in women as it does in men.

Determination and Perseverance in Pursuing Goals

Not only does DHEA, through its conversion to testosterone, help maintain physical energy and muscle mass, it also affects behavioral traits also linked to male hormone production, such as assertiveness and the maintenance of libido.

Assertiveness and sex drive are, of course, as important to women as they are to men in enhancing the quality of our lives and DHEA seems to provide real benefits in this regard. For this reason, it is important in supporting the ability to pursue goals.

One of my patients Larissa, a delightful woman in her sixties, was embarking on a new career as a counselor after having spent most of her active career life as a businesswoman. She was taking many courses in her newly chosen field but was finding it difficult to keep up with the class work and do her papers and exams. She found that she was "running out of steam" and lacked the energy and perseverance to keep up with her goals. A powerful program of nutritional supplementation and DHEA helped her greatly and she felt much of her assertiveness and drive return with this program.

The field of medicine is notoriously poor at restoring functional qualities such as physical energy, vitality, and stamina in individuals who may be losing these capabilities. Supplementation with DHEA should be considered for individuals who are losing these attributes.

While I recommend seeing a physician before starting DHEA supplementation, this is not always possible, as many areas lack physicians who have any experience using the newer hormone therapies like DHEA. As a result, millions of units are currently being sold on a self-medication basis.

If you elect to use DHEA without a physician's guidance, buy the lowest-dose products available in your health food store or pharmacy, begin to use it cautiously, and do not go above 25 mg on your own. Let your physician recommend dosages at higher levels, and be sure to carefully monitor the effects on your body. I discuss this in more detail in chapter 7.

The Ability to Remain Calm Under Pressure

Animal studies suggest that DHEA may have a modulating effect on stress hormones, thereby lessening the impact of stress on the body. This response involves an increase in the production of stress hormones, or corticosteroids. DHEA can lessen the intensity of this response so that corticosteroid levels do not increase as dramatically. This benefit was found in a study on mice, published in *Pharmacology, Biochemistry and Behavior*. The researchers concluded that DHEA has anxiety-reducing properties.

In humans, DHEA also appears to reduce levels of fear and anxiety lined to stress. DHEA helps to create more of a sense of peace and calmness when dealing with stress inducing situations.

However, it appears that stress itself can lower levels of DHEA. Amazingly, this is true in younger people, not just older women and men who would be more vulnerable to diminished DHEA levels.

This has been shown in several studies. In one notable study, appearing in the *European Journal of Endocrinology,* a group of eighteen Norwegian cadets were given a five-day military training course. They participated in continuous heavy physical activities and had almost no food or sleep. DHEA-S blood levels were measured for ten of the cadets at the start of the test and at completion.

During the five days, the normal hourly changes in DHEA output were diminished, and while DHEA levels did increase with continued stress, once the training was over, DHEA-S levels remained low during the recovery period.

According to another study, appearing in *Experimental and Clinical Endocrinology*, levels of DHEA in patients undergoing thyroid surgery continued to decline during the two days following the operation.

This decline in DHEA levels can lead to a situation in which stress hormones dominate. Older persons are more likely to experience this oversensitivity to stress hormones, as they are in a period of their lives where DHEA levels naturally decline. In a study appearing in the *Journal of Clinical Endocrinology and Metabolism*, researchers measured DHEA and cortisol levels in sixty-two volunteers, aged three to eighty-five, and found that the ratio of cortisol to DHEA in the brain increased with age. High levels of cortisol are known to cause brain damage in animals and humans. This imbalance of cortisol to DHEA may permit normal levels of cortisol to become toxic.

Optimism and Vision

Many individuals and studies report that DHEA has the ability to enhance psychological well-being, a state of mind in which all seems right with the world. A small but significant study cited in an article appearing in the Lancet found that when volunteers were given 50 mg per day of DHEA, 70 percent of them reported an increase in feelings of well-being. At the same time, DHEA helps alleviate depression.

A study appearing in *Biological Psychiatry* observed the effects of DHEA on older patients. The dosage was 30 to 60 mg a day of oral DHEA, given for four weeks. Ratings for depression significantly declined, but when treatment stopped, measurements of mood returned to pretreatment levels.

Having a sense of well-being predisposes a person to having an optimistic approach to life and encourages visionary thinking. Because DHEA fosters this general state of mind, having higher levels of DHEA may allow an individual to live a fuller life.

This is indicated by a study published in the *Journal of Clinical Epidemiology*. In this study volunteers, aged 70 to 79, were assembled into three groups representing various levels of functioning- high, medium and low functioning, reflecting the quality of their lives.

Not surprisingly, the values of DHEA-S increased with functional levels, from a value of forty-eight in the low group to sixty-nine in the top group. Persons in the highest-functioning group felt more effective, had a greater sense of mastery, and were more satisfied with life. Furthermore, these individuals also engaged in more productive activities, exercised more, and engaged more frequently in volunteer activities. This is a terrific reflection on how beneficial higher levels of DHEA are in helping to maintain a satisfying quality of life.

4

DHEA and Your Health

DHEA provides remarkable support to the body and healing benefits for a wide range of physical ailments. The research in this area is very widespread in terms of the areas examined. In this chapter, I discuss these positive findings. You may find support for the use of DHEA for health issues that you are currently trying to find solutions for.

Menopausal Symptoms

As estrogen production declines in menopause, many women experience a variety of symptoms due to this deficiency. Supplementing with DHEA can help remedy these complaints. Once it is absorbed, DHEA is converted to estrone, a form of estrogen, so DHEA supplementation can become a natural form of estrogen therapy for many women.

During meno-pause, women may experience a thinning of the vaginal tissue and a decline in vaginal secretions. At this time in life, a woman's skin becomes drier. DHEA has been found to revive vaginal tissues; it also activates oil glands in the skin, restoring a youthful texture to the hands and face. It can help to relieve insomnia and many of the emotional stress symptoms that often become more prevalent in women who are in midlife and beyond.

Lorraine was 70 years old when she came to see me. She had always been very strong and healthy. However, after entering menopause, she experienced mild to moderate hot flashes for many years. She tried conventional HRT on and off for nearly 10 years, but kept discontinuing it because she did not like the negative side effects she was experiencing.

Lorraine consulted me because she felt like the "wheels were beginning to come off." She complained of increasing stiffness in her fingers, hips, and knees; some loss of short-term memory; and not quite as much energy as she had had in previous years. She was also concerned about her risk of breast disease.

The combination of her age and her symptoms made Lorraine a good candidate for DHEA, along with a strong, hormone-supportive program.

Balance Thyroid Levels

According to a study from Clinical Chemistry, DHEA levels may affect the levels of thyroid hormone in your body. Researchers found that 24 patients with hypothyroidism (low thyroid function) had significantly lower levels of DHEA than those found in the healthy participants.

Similarly, 22 participants with hyperthyroidism (high thyroid function) also had significantly elevated levels of DHEA as compared to the healthy patients. Thus, maintaining healthy, balanced DHEA levels appears to be helpful in supporting healthy thyroid function.

Stress and Anxiety

The natural stress-reducing aspect of DHEA is another one of its amazing benefits. Animal studies suggest that DHEA may have a modulating effect on stress hormones, thereby lessening the impact of stress on the body. The stress response involves an increase in the production of stress hormones, or corticosteroids. DHEA can lessen the strength of this stress response so that corticosteroid levels do not increase as dramatically. This can be extremely beneficial for women in menopause that are suffering from the brain and nervous system related changes that occur during this time of life.

Depression

As I discussed in the previous chapter, many individuals and studies report that DHEA has the ability to enhance psychological well-being, a state of mind in which all seems right with the world. Having a sense of wellbeing predisposes a person to having an optimistic approach to life and encourages visionary thinking. Because DHEA fosters this general state of mind, having higher levels of DHEA may allow an individual to live a fuller, more positive and enjoyable life.

Insomnia

DHEA plays a role in reducing fatigue by improving the quality of sleep. Women with insufficient levels of DHEA often miss out on this crucial benefit. They can experience either difficulty falling asleep or staying asleep. Fortunately, supplementing with DHEA has been shown to be effective in treating insomnia.

A study published in the *American Journal of Physiology* demonstrated that a single 500 mg oral dose of DHEA significantly increased rapid eye movement (REM) sleep in ten healthy young men. This phase of sleep, when most dreaming occurs, is essential for a person to feel rested. While this is an enormous dose of DHEA, much greater than that normally used in clinical practice, the finding in this study may have important implications in the field of sleep physiology. Obviously, much more research needs to be done in this area before DHEA can be definitively recommended as a sleep-enhancing therapy.

Loss of Libido

Not only does DHEA help maintain physical energy and muscle mass through its conversion to testosterone, it also affects behavioral traits linked to male hormone production, such as assertiveness and the maintenance of libido. Specifically, I have found DHEA to be useful not only for men with loss of libido but also for women. This is definitely a benefit of DHEA that has been reported by many patients using this hormone.

Mika, a 51-year-old office manager, consulted me for treatment of her perimenopausal symptoms. As her periods began to be lighter and more irregular, she also found that her sex drive began to diminish. She had a high-stress diet. She drank too much red wine and ate too much white-flour pasta with butter and cream sauces. She definitely needed to start eating a healthier diet, to which she reluctantly agreed. She also started a nutritional supplement program that included DHEA.

After a few weeks on this program, her interest in sex returned, and she became a more enthusiastic participant in sexual activity with her husband.

Poor Memory and Mental Fog

Having a good memory is one of the most fundamental skills required in all areas of life. And there is both anecdotal and scientific evidence that DHEA enhances memory. DHEA improves the brain's ability to process and store information. In a study published in *Biological Psychiatry*, six middle-aged and elderly volunteers were monitored for the effects of DHEA supplementation on memory. For four weeks, the volunteers were given 30 to 90 mg a day of oral DHEA so that the hormone was restored to youthful levels. The researchers noted a significant improvement in memory performance.

The mechanism by which DHEA may benefit memory is not known. However, DHEA has been added to tissue cultures of brain cells from mice, which has stimulated the growth of certain structures that allow communication between nerves. Older mice injected with DHEA completed a memory test as easily as younger mice and retained this information at a second testing.

In yet another study, various individual steroid horm-ones were administered to mice that were given a shock-avoidance test. In this instance, DHEA was able to enhance learning in doses 10 to 100 times lower than those of other steroid hormones.

People taking DHEA find that it aids two specific types of memory: (1) incidental memory, the ability to recall details of recent events, and (2) semantic memory, the ability to retrieve more general types of stored data.

These two types of memory tend to decline with age and are the first aspects of memory to deteriorate in patients with Alzheimer's disease. Various studies have been conducted to discover whether DHEA may be useful in treating Alzheimer's. Current research is focusing on the most effective dosages and on whether DHEA is best used in the early stages of the disease.

Osteoporosis

Osteoporosis and osteopenia are so prevalent in women today, it is critical to find and use safe, natural therapies that can help to support bone mass. Unfortunately, thinning bones are another common occurrence associated with menopause and low levels of estrogen, as well as progesterone and testosterone.

There is much research surrounding the effectiveness of DHEA on bone health. Animal studies have found that DHEA increases bone mineral density. Human studies are also showing that DHEA can increase bone mineral density at various bone sites. One such study from the *Journal of Clinical Endocrinology and Metabolism* found that DHEA supplementation improved bone density.

Researchers gave 70 women and 70 men aged 60 to 88 years old either 50 mg of DHEA or a placebo every day for one year. They found that those participants taking DHEA had significantly greater bone mineral density in their hips, thigh bone (femoral shaft), and top of thigh bone (trochanter). The women taking

DHEA also enjoyed greater bone density in their lower back (lumbar spine).

A study from the *New England Journal of Medicine* had similar results. Researchers evaluated the effect of DHEA supplementation on elderly women and men. They found that of the eight bone sites they tested (mostly spine, hip, thigh, and wrist), DHEA significantly increased bone mineral density at the wrist in women and the femoral neck (where the hip connects to the thigh) in men.

There was also an increase in three other sites in those people taking DHEA. Of the three remaining bone sites tested, two others also showed a slight increase in bone mineral density in those participants taking DHEA.

In other words, DHEA supplementation significantly improved bone health in two bone sites, was helpful in five others, and was of no benefit in just one site tested. Clearly, the use of DHEA can help to improve bone mineral density.

This is very important news for women, given the significant problems and side effects of both conventional hormone replacement therapy and drugs used to treat osteoporosis and osteopenia.

Cardiovascular Disease

Heart disease is currently the leading cause of death among Americans. In younger women, coronary-heart disease (CHD) is rare, but by the time a woman reaches age 65, her probability of having the disease is equal to that of a man.

Healthy levels of DHEA appear to be protective. The majority of research studies on this topic support the conclusion that maintaining healthy levels of DHEA can help prevent heart disease. Conversely, depressed levels of DHEA can be a risk factor for heart disease. An article appearing in the *Journal of Internal Medicine* referred to a study conducted in Poland in which women with coronary heart disease had significantly lower levels of DHEA-S than women with no heart disease.

Many theories of how DHEA protects against heart disease are now being investigated. Both laboratory and human studies have indicated that DHEA helps prevent blood clots that can block an artery and trigger a heart attack or stroke. DHEA is known to reduce plaque on the walls of arteries, which can also limit blood flow. In an animal study published in the *Journal of Clinical Investigation*, rabbits with severe atherosclerosis were treated with DHEA, and plaque size was reduced by almost 50 percent. It has also been observed that women taking DHEA experience a decline in cholesterol levels. DHEA may produce this effect by facilitating the breakdown of cholesterol in the liver.

In a healthy person, DHEA is able to counteract these risk factors for heart disease. But various conditions, such as stress, can lower DHEA levels and increase the probability of cardiac problems. As mentioned in the previous chapter, DHEA can greatly reduce the stress response in susceptible people.

High levels of the hormone insulin, which manages the metabolism and storage of sugars and starches, can also reduce DHEA levels. To maintain cardiovascular health, there needs to be a balance between these two powerful hormones. During the early stages of diabetes, insulin levels rise and DHEA activity is blocked.

This was observed in a study published in the *FASEB Journal*. The researchers observed that insulin lowers blood concentrations of DHEA and DHEA-S by decreasing production of these hormones and by increasing their breakdown and excretion.

They suggested that the well-known association between high levels of insulin in the blood (hyperinsulinemia) and heart disease may be through insulin's effect on DHEA. Gaining a great deal of weight, as well as normal aging, is also associated with increased insulin levels. In this way, both obesity and aging can also lower DHEA.

Excess Weight

As people age, their weight can slowly increase to a condition of obesity. As the excess pounds and fat accumulate, self-esteem can plummet, and health problems such as heart disease and diabetes are more likely to occur. It appears that levels of DHEA influence the changes in weight and body composition that occur over time.

There is conflicting evidence about whether DHEA promotes weight loss, but certain animal studies indicate this is possible. In one such study, published in the *International Journal of Obesity*, nineteen dogs were given increasing doses of DHEA daily. Over the six months of the study, 68 percent of these animals lost an average of 3 percent of their total body weight each month, without any reduction in food intake. This suggests that DHEA may affect metabolism, the process by which food is turned into energy, causing more calories to be used.

There is even clearer evidence that DHEA causes fat to be replaced with muscle. One study, published in the *Journal of Clinical Endocrinology and Metabolism*, monitored ten men for body fat. The men, in their early twenties and matched for weight, were divided into two groups. One group was treated with DHEA, a 400 mg dosage four times a day for twenty-eight days, and the other group was left untreated. The men reported no changes in their regular act-ivities or diet.

At the end of the treatment period, it was found that among the five men receiving DHEA, their average percentage of body fat dropped 31 percent. However, there was no drop in weight, suggesting that while there was a decline in fat, muscle mass increased. No change in these measurements occurred in the untreated men. Similar changes in women in terms of building muscle mass may find support, too since DHEA converts to testosterone as well as estrogen in women.

Some researchers suggest that DHEA may decrease body fat by blocking the synthesis of fatty acids, which eventually become body fat. Others have noted that DHEA can act as an appetite suppressant and dampen the desire for fatty foods. As the DHEA story unfolds, dieters may someday find that DHEA can help them toward the goal of having a fitter, healthier, slimmer body.

Diabetes

Every woman should be aware of the increasing incidence of diabetes in the Western world. Once this disease has been diagnosed, it often has very dramatic effects that can negatively affect your health, quality of life, and even your longevity. Prevention and effective treatments, including

DHEA, are key to fending off diabetes and keeping your blood sugar levels low.

Blood sugar (glucose) is a source of energy used throughout the body. Normally, the pancreas produces a sufficient amount of insulin, the hormone that manages levels of glucose in the blood and enables the storage of glucose in the cells. The balance between insulin activity and cell uptake determines blood sugar levels. As a person ages, the cells become less responsive to insulin and do not store glucose as readily, a condition called insulin resistance.

However, studies have shown that DHEA causes tissues to be more insulin sensitive. In this way, DHEA may one day become a useful treatment for diabetes (a disease characterized by high levels of insulin and glucose circulating in the blood, coupled with insulin resistance of the cells).

In addition, as insulin levels increase, the amount of DHEA-S decreases, according to a study published in the *Journal of Clinical Endocrinology*. This was observed in non-diabetic men who were treated with a medication that lowers circulating insulin.

Weakened Immune Function

A compromised immune system often leads to prolonged colds and infection, stress and strain in the body, and impaired hormonal function. By working at the cellular level, DHEA can positively impact immune function.

A variety of laboratory studies, both animal and human, give evidence of DHEA's role in immunity. One such study, appearing in *the Journal of Steroid Biochemistry and Molecular Biology*, analyzed the amount of DHEA by-products present in various tissues in mice. The results suggested that in tissues involved in the immune response, locally produced DHEA metabolites, or breakdown products, may participate in the regulation of the immune response.

Health care practitioners working with DHEA find that patients with adequate levels tend not to have colds or the flu. But there is also indication that DHEA may be a potent tool for combating diseases directly involved with the immune system itself. These include autoimmune diseases such as rheumatoid arthritis, multiple sclerosis, ulcerative colitis, and lupus. There is also evidence that DHEA can be of benefit in the treatment of AIDS (which is caused by the human immunodeficiency virus).

A study published in *the Journal of Infectious Diseases* measured levels of DHEA in forty-one men who were asymptomatic HIV-seropositive who subsequently progressed to AIDS. They also monitored DHEA in forty-one similar men who did not develop AIDS, and in an equal number of men who were

HIV-1-seronegative. The researchers found that among the men who developed AIDS, DHEA levels were lower than in the other two groups five months before progression to AIDS.

How DHEA levels impact immunity involves changes that occur in the immune system with age. In the immune system, the fighter T cells identify and disarm invading substances that find their way into the body. One type of T cell is the suppressor cell, which detects which substances are foreign versus which ones are a natural part of body tissues. With age, suppressor cells perform these functions less efficiently. DHEA may help prevent this decline and even reverse it.

Another component of the immune system is cytokines. These are hormone-like substances, produced by immune cells that determine how our cells respond. Cytokines can either trigger a reaction or inhibit one, and either promote or limit growth. They are the communication system between immune system cells. With age, however, they begin to send the wrong messages. It appears that DHEA may restore their proper function.

Lastly, DHEA suppresses the stress response, which can weaken the immune system and cause a person to be vulnerable to disease. Low levels of stress hormones are associated with higher levels of DHEA.

As a physician, I have seen many women whose weak immunity results in chronic and recurrent infections. These women are often miserable because of the havoc that these infections are causing in their lives. I have seen women who were experiencing colds and bronchial symptoms on a monthly or even biweekly basis as well as women whose digestive symptoms from bacterial and parasitic invasions were causing frequent indigestion and diarrhea, to give but a few examples. Low levels of DHEA were dragging down their immunity along with other risk factors.

There is also indication that DHEA may be a potent tool for combatting diseases directly involved with the immune system itself. These include autoimmune diseases such as rheumatoid arthritis, systemic lupus multiple sclerosis, erythematosus, and ulcerative colitis. Supplementation with DHEA may be very beneficial for women who are suffering from autoimmune conditions.

Asthma

Studies have found that persons with asthma have lower levels of DHEA. Various medications are used to treat the tightening and spasming of the lung tubes (bronchi). It has been noted that when a medication such as prednisone (a potent anti-inflammatory agent) is given to asthma patients, DHEA-S levels rise.

Cancer

Research has shown that individuals who develop certain kinds of cancer have low levels of DHEA. A retrospective study, published in *Cancer Research*, compared thirty-five individuals who developed bladder cancer with sixty-nine others who remained cancer-free. The cancer patients had significantly lower levels of DHEA and DHEA-S.

Another study, of 37 lung cancer patients at the Gujarat Cancer and Research Institute, in Ahmedabad, India, found that these patients also had lower levels of DHEA-S, as compared with the control group; the research was published in *Neoplasma*.

It is also known that levels of DHEA are significantly lower in patients with both breast cancer in women and prostate cancer in men. This is particularly significant because both breast and prostate cancer are very common cancers in women and men.

Various laboratory and animal studies suggest that DHEA protects against a wide range of carcinogens and may inhibit the growth of tumors. Whether the initiating carcinogenic substance is cigarette smoke, heavy metals such as lead and cadmium, or radiation, DHEA may be able to block its activation.

One theory is that DHEA blocks an enzyme required for certain cancer-promoting chemical reactions to occur. DHEA may also prevent the formation of free radicals, which are unstable atoms that easily bond to other atoms. Free radicals can damage cells and cause them to mutate, resulting in cancerous growth.

5

Testing for DHEA Deficiency

DHEA is produced in abundance by your body during youth, but its production slows markedly with time. To begin to determine whether your body's supply of this hormone has lessened enough to affect your ability to perform at your best and maintain optimal health, see the following checklist. If you answer yes to four or more of these questions, you very likely need to increase your DHEA levels.

DHEA Deficiency Checklist
- I am over the age of 50.
- I experience symptoms of menopause such as hot flashes.
- I have low libido.
- I suffer from insomnia.
- I am unable to handle stress.
- I am easily upset.
- I have a negative outlook on life.
- I am often unable to recall details of recent events.
- I have a history of osteoporosis or osteopenia (low bone mass).
- I have a history of cardiovascular disease.

- I have significant excess body fat.
- I am at risk for diabetes.
- I have a history of autoimmune disease, including rheumatoid arthritis, lupus, multiple sclerosis, ulcerative colitis, and/or AIDS.
- I have a weak immune system and am prone to colds and flu.
- I am at high risk for cancer, especially bladder cancer.
- I suffer from asthma.
- I lack muscle mass and strength.
- I tend to tire easily; my level of stamina is low.

If your responses suggest that your DHEA level is low, then your next step is to get your hormone levels tested.

Testing for DHEA Deficiency

The DHEA in the blood is a combination of DHEA sulfate (DHEA-S) and unbound, or free, DHEA. It is generally thought that unbound DHEA is most active and that DHEA-S is not fully metabolically active. Therefore, it is important that any lab assessment distinguish between the two. When a physician is assessing a patient's DHEA levels in relation to specific illnesses, this differentiation takes on special meaning. For instance, research has shown that DHEA levels, but not levels of DHEA-S, can be predictive of the progression of HIV to AIDS.

Levels of DHEA are routinely assessed using a blood test, but salivary testing is also thought to be accurate. DHEA can also be assessed using a 24-hour urine test. If you are taking DHEA supplementation, you need to have initial levels tested and then be tested again every few months, to keep the amount in the upper normal range typical of a young person.

Ranges of DHEA Levels

As supplementing with DHEA is a relatively new practice, it is a particularly good idea to have levels monitored regularly. However, some physicians believe that this is unnecessary when the dosages used are low. A cautious approach is also advised to monitor metabolites of DHEA such as androsterone and etiocholanolone, as well as hormone metabolites such as testosterone. This can be done using a 24-hour urine test. Some practitioners also think it is important to monitor DHEA levels if an individual has a significant illness and that at age 40, all people should obtain a baseline reading.

Range of DHEA blood levels in adult women:

130 to 980 ng/dl

Range of DHEA-S blood levels in adult women:

Aged 31-50: 2 to 379 µg/dl
Postmenopausal: 30 to 260 µg/dl

Range of DHEA salivary levels in women:

40 to 140 pg/ml

If your results indicate that you are deficient in DHEA (or if you scored high on the checklist), then the next chapter is a must-read. You'll discover how you can restore your DHEA levels quickly and effectively.

6

Support Your Own Production of DHEA

In this chapter, I'll share with you my exciting program to help you restore and maintain proper DHEA levels within your own body. I discuss how you can restore this critical hormone at the central nervous system level with the help of key neurotransmitters and glandulars, as well as some powerful herbs.

Since the vast majority of DHEA is produced in your adrenals (with small amounts in your ovaries), you'll also learn about key vitamins and nutrients that help to keep your DHEA levels in the healthy range by optimizing adrenal and ovarian function.

Let's get started!

Boost Your Adrenal Function

Because so much of DHEA's production takes place in the adrenals, with a little also made in the ovaries, it is critical that you keep these glands operating at peak performance. The best way to accomplish this is to use specific nutrients that support functioning at the central nervous system level, as well as the ovarian and adrenal level.

Support Production from the Central Nervous System

As with all the sex hormones, production begins in your brain. We've been traditionally taught that human beings have one brain that is divided into many different parts. But more and more research is putting the "one brain" idea to the test. In fact, it's starting to be widely accepted that the human skull actually houses not one brain, but three—the reptilian brain, the limbic brain, and the neocortical brain.

The reptilian brain is the oldest part of the brain. It controls basic bodily functions like heart rate, breathing, body temperature, hunger, and fight-or-flight responses. Basic drives and instincts, such as defending territory and keeping safe from harm, are other functions of the reptilian brain. The structures in the brain that perform these functions are the brain stem (which controls breathing, heart rate, and blood pressure) and the cerebellum (which controls movement, balance, and posture).

The limbic, or mammalian, brain developed once mammals started roaming the earth. It includes the amygdala, which controls memory and emotions; the hippocampus, which controls memories and learning; and the hypothalamus, which controls emotions (among many other things). Therefore, the limbic brain allows mammals to learn, retain memories, and show emotions.

The neocortical brain, or neocortex, is the complex maze of grey matter that surrounds the reptilian and limbic brains, and accounts for about 85 percent of brain mass. It is found in the brains of primates and humans, and is responsible for sensory perception, abstract thought, imagination, and consciousness. It also controls language, social interactions, and higher communication.

The Chemistry of the Brain

Like the three parts of the brain, there are also three key types of brain chemicals: neuropeptides, neurohormones, and neurotransmitters.

Neuropeptides are responsible for the cell-to-cell communication system in your body. A peptide is a short chain of amino acids connected together, and a neuropeptide is a peptide found in neural tissue.

Neuropeptides are widespread in the central and peripheral nervous systems and different neuropeptides have different excitatory or inhibitory actions.

Neuropeptides control such a diverse array of functions in the body. When they work together properly, the wonderful results in your body include elevated mood and other positive behaviors and emotions, stronger bones, better resistance to disease, glowing skin and boosted metabolism. Conversely, if your neuropeptides function abnormally, the result can be an increased tendency towards neurological and mental disorders such as Alzheimer's disease, epilepsy and schizophrenia.

There are several types of neuropeptides. The most common include endorphins and beta-endorphins. Endorphins are opioid peptides, meaning they have morphine-like effects within the body. They produce feelings of well-being and euphoria, and a rush of endorphins can lead to feelings of exhilaration brought on by pain, danger, or stress. Endorphins also may also play a role in memory, sexual activity, and body temperature.

Beta-endorphins are another form of opioid peptides, but they are stronger than endorphins. They are composed of 31 amino acids and work in the body by numbing pain, increasing relaxation, and promoting a general feeling of well-being.

While there are many hormones and hormonal interactions that occur in the brain and body, the most widely known neurohormone is melatonin. Melatonin is produced by the pineal gland and regulates our patterns of sleep.

Neurotransmitters are naturally occurring chemicals that relay electrical messages between nerve cells throughout your body. While all three types of neurochemicals are important for hormone and overall health, neurotransmitters are very important for the production of sex hormones.

In the aggregate, all three types of neurochemicals help to regulate the brain's endocrine glands, specifically the hypothalamus and pituitary gland. The hypothalamus is the master endocrine gland contained within your brain that regulates your production of sex hormones. This gland produces a precursor hormone called gonadotropin releasing hormone (GnRH).

The neurotransmitters norepinephrine, epinephrine, dopamine, and serotonin regulate the hypothalamus' release of GnRH. Without proper production and balance of these neurotransmitters, you cannot have proper production and balance of the sex hormones either, including the production of DHEA as well as the hormones that depend on adequate production of DHEA, testosterone and estrogen.

To ensure that neurotransmitter production is being properly supported, and that the neurotransmitters themselves are supporting the production of hormones by the pituitary glands, you need adequate amounts of precursor amino acids such as tyrosine, phenylalanine, and 5-HTP.

All neurotransmitters fall into one of two pathways that help to support your overall health and well-being. The first leads to the production of the inhibitory neurotransmitter serotonin, while the second leads to the production of the excitatory neurotransmitters dopamine, norepinephrine, and epinephrine.

Generally speaking, the inhibitory neurotransmitters quiet down the processes of your body, while the excitatory neurotransmitters speed them up. Thus, the brain chemicals produced through these two pathways oppose and complement one another. Within your brain, serotonin often inhibits the firing of neurons, which dampens many of your behaviors. In fact, serotonin acts as a kind of chemical restraint system.

Of all your body's chemicals, serotonin has one of the most widespread effects on the brain and physiology. It plays a key role in regulating temperature, blood pressure, blood clotting, immunity, pain, digestion, sleep, and biorhythms. Along with another inhibitory neurotransmitter, GABA (gamma-aminobutyric acid) serotonin also produces a relaxing effect on your mood. Taurine, a type of amino acid, is often used in a similar fashion as these two neurotransmitters because it also has therapeutic, inhibitory effects on your body.

Dopamine, norepinephrine, and epinephrine make up the excitatory neurotransmitter pathway. Glutamate is an important excitatory neurotransmitter, though it is not part of this pathway. Unlike serotonin, which has a relaxing effect on your energy and behavior, excitatory neurotransmitters energize and elevate your mood. In addition to their powerful anti-depressant effects, they support alertness, optimism, motivation, zest for life, and sex drive.

In order to ensure that you have adequate neurotransmitter levels for healthy hormone production, you need to supplement with key amino acids, vitamins, and minerals. All neurotransmitters are produced from amino acids found in the protein that you eat. The essential amino acid tryptophan is initially converted into an intermediary substance called 5-hydroxytryptophan (5-HTP), which is then converted into serotonin.

While tryptophan is available as a supplement and is abundant in turkey, pumpkin seeds, and almonds, I've found that 5-HTP is a more effective and reliable option for boosting your neurotransmitter production. Numerous double-blind studies have shown that 5-HTP is as effective as many of the more common antidepressant drugs and is associated with fewer and much milder side effects. In addition to increasing serotonin levels, 5-HTP triggers an increase in endorphins and other neurotransmitters that are often low in cases of depression.

The excitatory neurotransmitters are derived from tyrosine, an amino acid produced from the essential amino acid phenylalanine. A variety of vitamins and minerals, such as vitamin C, vitamin B6, and magnesium, act as co-factors and are necessary for the conversion of these amino acids into neurotransmitters.

To maintain proper serotonin levels, it is helpful to take 50-100 mg of 5-HTP once or twice a day, with one of the dosages taken at bedtime. Be sure to start at 50 mg and increase as necessary. If needed during the day, use carefully, as too much serotonin can interfere with your ability to drive or concentrate.

To maintain optimum dopamine levels, take 500-1,000 mg of tyrosine per day. Be sure to take in divided doses, half in the morning and half in the afternoon. Do not take in the evening, as it may interfere with sleep.

As I recommend with all nutritional supplements, you should start at the lower to more moderate dosage, such as 500 mg a day of tyrosine and 50 mg a day of 5-HTP. Stay on this dosage for two weeks. If you don't notice a reduction in your symptoms, gradually increase the dosage by 500 mg for tyrosine and 50 mg for 5-HTP every two weeks until you have either noticed a reduction in your symptoms or have reached the maximum dosages. I generally don't recommend going over 1,000 mg a day of tyrosine, although you may find that you need as much as 100-200 mg of 5-HTP once or even several times a day.

Additionally, be sure to use a high potency multi-vitamin mineral nutritional supplement so that you are taking in all of the co-factors needed to produce neurotransmitters. These include vitamin C, vitamin B6, folic acid, niacin, magnesium, and copper.

Note: I strongly advise that you undertake a program to restore, build and properly balance your neuro-transmitter levels under the care of a complementary physician, naturopath, or nutritionist. You should also have your neurotransmitter levels tested regularly, as dosage needs for the amino acids I have described often vary from woman to woman.

Test Your Neurotransmitter Levels

State-of-the-art neurotransmitter testing is currently available and can accurately pinpoint your exact levels of these essential brain chemicals. A leader in the development of neurotransmitter testing is NeuroScience, Inc., (888-342-7272 or neurorelief.com). They have developed sensitive testing for these neurochemicals that can be done through your urine. The test is simple to do, non-invasive, and can be done in the privacy of your own home. In addition to

NeuroScience, there are many other similar laboratories that offer neurotransmitter testing.

I would strongly recommend that you consider such testing if you suspect that you suffer from a moderate to severe neurotransmitter deficiency. Your health care provider will need to order these tests for you.

Support Production in the Ovaries and Adrenals

You now know that hormone stimulation begins in your brain via the neurotransmitters and your brain's endocrine glands. However, the actual production of DHEA takes place primarily in your adrenal glands and ovaries. For this reason, it is crucial that you keep these glands healthy so they can function at peak performance. To do this, you need to make sure you have adequate amounts of the following nutrients: glandulars, beta-carotene, vitamin C, vitamin B5, zinc, and magnesium.

Glandular Therapy

Many women have had great success with the use of glandular therapy. Glandulars are purified extracts from the secretory endocrine glands of animals, usually the thyroid and adrenal glands, as well as the thymus, pituitary, pancreas, and ovaries.

In the past, most experts believed that glandulars could not be effective because the intestinal lining of a healthy person was impenetrable, and that proteins and large peptides could not breach its barrier.

However, recent evidence has shown that large macromolecules can and do pass completely intact from the intestinal tract into the bloodstream. In fact, there's further evidence to suggest that your body is able to determine which molecules it needs to absorb whole, and which can be broken down.

Both animal and human studies alike have proven this theory. In some cases, several whole proteins taken orally, including critical enzymes, have been shown to be absorbed intact into the bloodstream. Additionally, many smaller proteins and numerous hormones have also been found to be absorbed intact into the bloodstream, including thyroid, cortisone, and even insulin.

In essence, it means that the active properties of the glandulars stay active and intact, and are not destroyed in the digestive process. This is key to the success of glandular therapy, and explains why they clearly help to restore hormone function by supporting the health of your endocrine glands themselves.

There are multi and single-glandular systems available from a company like Standard Process, a leader in the field. However, they do require a prescription from a health care practitioner. Other good products are also available in health food stores and can be used as part of a nutritional program to support healthy menstruation.

One of the most widely used and accepted glandulars is for your adrenal glands. Whole adrenal gland preparations are not only beneficial in treating stress and fatigue, they have been shown to possess cortisone-like properties that help treat asthma, eczema, rheumatoid arthritis, and even psoriasis. They have also been found to help restore the health and function of compromised adrenal glands.

In one research study, eight women suffering from morning sickness (nausea and vomiting) who took oral adrenal cortex extract found relief within four days. A similar study gave both injected and oral adrenal cortex extract to 202 women also suffering from morning sickness. More than 85 percent of the women completely overcame their nausea and vomiting or showed significant improvement.

Another study looked at the use of adrenal glandulars to treat patients with chronic fatigue and immune dysfunction syndrome (CFIDS), as well as fibromyalgia. Researchers found that 5-13 mg of an adrenal glandular preparation significantly reduced pain and discomfort. Moreover, after six to 18 months, many of the patients were able to reduce and eventually discontinue treatment, while still enjoying relief.

Clearly glandulars work. To help support healthy DHEA levels, I suggest taking a good multi-glandular or single- glandular from a company like Standard Process. These could include glandulars such as adrenal, ovary, hypothalamus, and pituitary, depending on your specific needs. For an extra boost, you may also want to focus on adrenal and ovarian support specifically. I also recommend that you consider taking a whole brain glandular, if appropriate.

Nutritional Support for Hormone Production

In addition to glandular therapy, there are several important nutrients that are critical to the health of your adrenal glands. By supporting the function of the adrenals, these important nutrients ensure the proper production and balance of adrenal hormones, especially DHEA.

Beta-carotene is the plant-based, water-soluble precursor to vitamin A. It is very abundant in the adrenal glands and ovaries, and is essential for their healthy functioning. Beta-carotene is particularly plentiful in the corpus luteum of the ovary. After ovulation, the follicle that contained the egg that was expelled from the ovary during ovulation is then converted into a new structure called the corpus luteum.

The purpose of the corpus luteum is to switch from the estrogen production, which predominates during the first half of the menstrual cycle (days one to 14) to the production of progesterone and estrogen during the second half of your cycle (days 15 to 28). This is called the luteinizing process. Some research even suggests that a proper balance between carotene and the retinal form of vitamin A is necessary for proper luteal function.

To be sure that you have adequate amounts of vitamin A (as beta-carotene) in your system, I suggest taking 25,000-50,000 IU of beta-carotene a day. You can also eat foods rich in beta-carotene, such as spinach, squash, carrots, cantaloupe, pumpkin, and sweet potatoes.

Vitamin C is very well known for its cold- and flu-fighting properties, but most people don't realize that it is an integral part of the structure and function of the adrenal glands. Your adrenal glands have the highest concentration of vitamin C in your entire body. They use the vitamin to synthesize a variety of hormones and neurotransmitters. These include norepinephrine, epinephrine, and serotonin.

Furthermore, the adrenals use vitamin C to produce cortisol, which is released in times of stress. In fact, studies have shown that when you are under extreme stress, your vitamin C stores are rapidly depleted.

This means that your entire body suffers when you have vitamin C deficiency due to acute stress, with your adrenal glands taking the biggest hit.

To make sure your body and adrenal glands have adequate amounts of vitamin C, take 1,000 -3,000 mg of a mineral-buffered vitamin C each day, in divided doses. Also increase your consumption of vitamin C-rich foods, including citrus fruits, strawberries, peaches, broccoli, tomatoes, and spinach.

B vitamins, especially B5 (pantothenic acid), play a crucial role in adrenal function. They are critical for stress management, neurotransmitter synthesis, and hormone regulation. In particular, B5 is the primary nourishing nutrient of your adrenal glands. It is necessary to stimulate the adrenal glands to begin hormone production. B5 is also needed to produce glucocorticoids, including cortisol. Not surprisingly, the symptoms of vitamin B5 deficiency—fatigue, headaches, sleep issues—mimic those of adrenal exhaustion.

For proper adrenal function, be sure to take 50-100 mg of a vitamin B-complex a day, with an additional 250-500 mg of B5 once or twice a day. You can also increase your intake of foods high in B vitamins, including liver, wheat germ, whole grains, legumes, egg yolks, salmon, royal jelly, sweet potatoes, and brewer's yeast.

Zinc not only supports healthy adrenal function, but it helps to produce testosterone and progesterone by promoting proper pregnenolone production. This essential trace mineral also helps in a variety of enzymatic functions, aids in vitamin A metabolism, and keeps your immune system strong.

To ensure that your adrenal glands have adequate amounts of zinc, I suggest taking 10-25 mg of zinc a day. You can also eat foods rich in zinc, such as oysters, pumpkin seeds, and eggs.

Magnesium is one of the basic building blocks needed by your adrenals to produce hormones. Adequate amounts of this essential mineral are also necessary to keep your adrenals balanced and functioning properly. Research has shown that low levels of magnesium can often indicate an overly stressed adrenal system. In fact, depressed and suicidal people have been found to be magnesium deficient.

You can maintain healthy adrenal function with 600-1000 mg of magnesium a day, as well as eating foods like meat, nuts, whole grains, and dairy, all of which are high in magnesium.

Nutrients to Lower Cortisol and Boost Adrenals

In addition to sex hormones such as DHEA, your adrenal glands also produce the stress hormone cortisol. When you are under extreme, chronic stress, your body pours out continual amounts of cortisol. Over time, this excess cortisol can lead to fatigue, weight gain, insomnia, low immune function, and even premature aging. In contrast, low levels of cortisol can indicate that your adrenal glands have become exhausted and are not functioning properly.

Fortunately, DHEA balances the effects of cortisol. In this way, DHEA helps you better deal with all forms of stress, be it physical, mental, or emotional. To this end, many herbs have been shown to improve DHEA levels by helping to lower cortisol and boost adrenal amounts of cortisol. I have used these herbs — namely Rhodiola rosea, panax ginseng, Siberian ginseng, and licorice root — as well as the vitamin PABA in my practice for many years, and many of my patients have found them to be effective remedies.

Rhodiola rosea has been used medicinally for nearly 2,000 years. The ancient Greeks revered this rose-like rootstock, as did Siberian healers, who believed that people who drank Rhodiola tea on a regular basis would live to be more than 100 years old.

Rhodiola works to support all hormone production by easing stress and fatigue. Both destroy adrenal function and healthy sex hormone production, including pregnenolone. According to the journal *Phytomedicine*, Rhodiola is particularly effective in fighting stress-induced fatigue. In one study, researchers tested 40 male medical students during exam time to determine if the herb positively affected physical fitness, as well as mental well-being and capacity.

The students were divided into 2 groups and given either 50 mg of Rhodiola rosea extract or placebo twice a day for 20 days. Researchers found that those students who took the extract had a significant decrease in mental fatigue and improved psycho-motor function, with a 50 percent improvement in neuromotor function. In addition, scores from exams taken immediately after the study showed that the extract group had an average grade of 3.47, as compared to 3.20 for the placebo group.

To ease fatigue, stress, or anxiety—all of which can play havoc with your pregnenolone production—I recommend taking 50-100 mg of Rhodiola rosea three times a day, standardized to 3 percent rosavins and 0.8 percent salidrosides. While the herb is generally considered safe, some reports have indicated that it may counteract the effects of anti-arrhythmic medications. Therefore, if you are currently taking this type of medication, I suggest you discuss the use of Rhodiola rosea with your physician.

Panax ginseng is an ivy-like ground cover originating in the wild, damp woodlands of northern China and Korea. It has been used in Chinese herbal medicine for more than 4,000 years. In colonial North America, ginseng was a major export product. The wild form is now rare, but panax ginseng is a widely cultivated plant.

Ginseng has a legendary status among herbs. Happily, enough good research exists to demonstrate ginseng's activity, especially when high-quality extracts, standardized for active components, are used.

High quality ginseng supports the strength and balance of our endocrine glands, thereby supporting the production of our sex hormones, including DHEA. Many of the symptoms linked to DHEA deficiency can be decreased with the use of ginseng.

Ginseng also has a balancing, tonic effect on the systems and organs of the body involved in the stress response. It contains at least 13 different saponins, a class of chemicals found in many plants, especially legumes, which take their name from their ability to form a soap-like froth when shaken with water. These compounds (triterpene glycosides) are the most pharmaceutically active constituents of ginseng. Saponins benefit hormone production, as well as cardiovascular function, immunity, and the central nervous system.

During times of stress, the saponins in the ginseng act on the hypothalamus and pituitary glands, increasing the release of adrenocorticotrophin, or ACTH (a hormone produced by the pituitary that promotes the manufacture and secretion of adrenal hormones). As a result, ginseng increases the release of adrenal cortisone and other adrenal hormones, and prevents their depletion from stress. Other substances associated with the pituitary are also released, such as endorphins. Ginseng is used to prevent adrenal atrophy, which can be a side effect of cortisone drug treatment. Ginseng's ability to support the health and function of the adrenal glands during times of stress, as well as the improved hormone health that occurs with the use of ginseng, clearly supports the production of DHEA itself by the adrenal glands.

In a study published in *Drugs Under Experimental and Clinical Research*, two groups of volunteers suffering from fatigue due to physical or mental stress were given nutritional supplementation over a 12-week period. One hundred sixty-three volunteers were given a multivitamin and multi mineral complex, and 338 volunteers received the same product, plus a standardized Chinese ginseng extract.

Once a month, the volunteers were asked to fill out a questionnaire during a scheduled visit with a physician. This questionnaire contained 11 questions that asked them to describe their current level of physical energy, stamina, sense of well-being, libido, and quality of sleep.

While both groups experienced similar improvement in their quality of life, by the second visit the group using the ginseng extract almost doubled their improvement, based on their responses, by the third and fourth visits. Thus, ginseng appears to improve many parameters of well-being in individuals experiencing significant physical and emotional stress, when it is added to a multi-vitamin and multi mineral complex.

There is also evidence that ACTH (the hormone that stimulates the adrenal cortex) and adrenal hormones, which ginseng stimulates, are known to bind to brain tissue, increasing mental activity during stress.

For maximum benefit, take a high-quality preparation, an extract of the main root of a plant that is six to eight years old, standardized for ginsenoside content and ratio. Companies manufacturing ginseng products may mention the age of the plants used in their products as a testimony to their products' quality. Take a 100 mg capsule twice a day. If this is too stimulating, especially before bedtime, take the second dose mid-afternoon, or take only the morning dose.

Women using ginseng should purchase either Chinese or American ginseng that is better for the female body. Avoid Korean Red Ginseng that is better suited for men and too heating for the female body.

The documented side effects of ginseng include nervousness, hypertension, morning diarrhea, skin problems, insomnia, and euphoria. It is important that a person taking ginseng monitor themselves for these symptoms.

Siberian ginseng (Eleutherococcus senticosus) is in the same family as panax ginseng, but the exact composition differs considerably. The most pharmacologically active constituents in Siberian ginseng are eleutherosides, some of which are similar in structure to the saponins contained in Asian ginseng. Siberian ginseng has been used in Asia for nearly 2,000 years to combat fatigue and increase endurance. The medicinal properties of this plant have been studied in Russia, with a number of clinical and experimental studies demonstrating that eleutherosides are adaptogenic, increasing resistance to stress and fatigue.

According to a review of clinical trials of more than 2,100 healthy human subjects, ranging in age from 19 to 72, published in Economic Medicinal Plant Research, Siberian ginseng reduces activation of the adrenal cortex in response to stress, an action useful in the alarm stage of the fight-or-flight response. It also helps lower blood pressure. In this same study, data indicated that the eleutherosides increased the subjects' ability to withstand adverse physical conditions including heat, noise, motion, an increase in workload, and exercise. There was also improved quality of work under stressful work conditions and improved athletic performance.

Herbalists have also long prescribed Siberian ginseng for chronic-fatigue syndrome. One way in which ginseng may be effective in this capacity is through its ability to facilitate the conversion of fat into energy, in both intense and moderate physical activity, sparing carbohydrates, and postponing the point at which a person may "hit the wall." This occurs when stored glucose is depleted and can no longer serve as a source of energy.

Siberian ginseng is also used to treat a variety of psychological disturbances, including insomnia, hypochondriasis, and various neuroses. The reason Siberian ginseng is effective may be its ability to balance stress hormones from the adrenals and neurotransmitters such as epinephrine, serotonin, and dopamine, all of which support healthy hormone production by the adrenal glands and ovaries, including DHEA.

Though Siberian ginseng has virtually no toxicity, individuals with fever, hypertonic crisis, or myocardial infarction are advised not to use it. A standard dosage of the fluid extract (33 percent ethanol) ranges from 3-5 ml, three times a day, for periods of up to 60 consecutive days. An equivalent dosage of dry powdered extract (containing at least one percent eleutheroside F) is 100-200 mg 3 times a day. Take in multiple-dose regimens with two to three weeks between courses.

Take Care When Choosing Ginseng.

I have had a number of patients over the years who have bought inexpensive ginseng, either as a root or in capsule form, expecting miraculous results, given ginseng's venerable reputation. Unfortunately, these cheaper grades of ginseng rarely, if ever, deliver the punch that individuals expect—that is, the chemical equivalent of an auxiliary set of adrenal glands, testicles, or ovaries.

I have seen some remarkable results with high-grade ginseng purchased from reputable Chinese pharmacists that sell top-of-the-line herbs or American companies selling herbs of equivalent quality. Given that the potency of the therapeutic chemicals takes many years to develop within the ginseng root, it is no surprise that with ginseng, you get what you pay for. If you have a serious interest in using ginseng, for its adaptogenic properties, I strongly suggest that you search out the reputable dealers.

Licorice root has been enjoyed over the centuries as a candy, but it is also an herb with medicinal properties, featured in the great recorded herbals for 4,000 years. Respected by the ancient Egyptians, licorice was among the treasured items archaeologists discovered (in great quantities) when they opened King Tut's tomb. Sometime around the year 1600, John Josselyn of Boston listed licorice as one of the "precious herbs" brought from England to colonial America.

Licorice is used to treat respiratory conditions, ulcers, urinary and kidney problems, fatty liver, hepatitis, and the inflammation of arthritis. Licorice root also exhibits hormone-like activity. The herb increases the half-life of cortisol (the adrenal stress hormone), inhibiting the breakdown of adrenal hormones by the liver. As a result, licorice is useful in reversing low cortisol conditions, and in helping the adrenal glands rest and restore their function.

A standard dosage is 1 to 2 g of powdered root or 450-600 mg in capsule form three times a day with meals. Licorice has activity similar to aldosterone, the adrenal hormone responsible for regulating water and electrolytes within the body. As a result, taking large doses of licorice (10 to 14 g of the crude herb) can lead to high blood pressure, water retention, and sodium and potassium imbalances. Licorice should not be taken by children under age two. Caution should be used with older children, pregnant and nursing women, and people over 65. Start with low dosages and increase the strength only if necessary.

PABA (para-aminobenzoic acid), a fat-soluble B vitamin, has been shown to safely and effectively slow down the breakdown of sex hormones, including DHEA, in the liver. Plus, PABA has been shown to increase libido!

Research has also shown that higher levels of PABA are associated with better mood and outlook, better vaginal lubrication, and improved sex drive, all of which are indicative of higher testosterone levels. And since testosterone is made from DHEA, it stands to reason that PABA may slow the breakdown of both testosterone and DHEA.

To help impede the breakdown of DHEA, I recommend taking 400-500 mg of PABA a day.

7

Bioidentical DHEA

Until 1996, DHEA was regulated by the FDA and required a doctor's prescription. Now DHEA can be purchased in health food stores, most drugstores, and by mail order. While DHEA has gained great popularity as its availability has increased, it continues to be considered an alternative therapy.

The majority of DHEA is produced in laboratories from diosgenin. Research on DHEA is far behind that of other sex hormones such as estrogen and testosterone. However, the studies that have been performed show great promise.

Using DHEA

Various preparations of DHEA are on the market, as well as yam extracts, which are sometimes purported to be a substitute for DHEA. It is important to understand the differences between these products. The conversion of the extract to DHEA can be achieved only in the laboratory, not in the human body. Therefore, natural yam extract, while it does have some of its own health benefits, does not increase blood levels of DHEA. This was confirmed in a study published in *Life Science*. Seven men and women, aged 65 to 82, were given yam extract for three weeks with no change in their DHEA level. In contrast, when the same group received 85 mg of DHEA a day, their blood levels of DHEA doubled.

Different delivery systems produce markedly different rates of assimilation and absorption of DHEA. Be careful not to overdose if you switch from one method to another. Also, most dosages you will read about are based on DHEA in capsule form. Use the information below as a guideline for using a different delivery system.

Capsules

The assimilation and absorption rate is between 30 and 50 percent, because the DHEA is first processed through the liver before going into the bloodstream. Higher absorption rates may be attained by opening a capsule and pouring the contents under the tongue; hold this for a minute or two before swallowing it.

Liquid Sublinguals

Assimilation and absorption rates run as high as 90-95 percent. This is because these are held under the tongue and the absorption is directly into the bloodstream, bypassing the liver. Sublinguals usually provide 5 mg of DHEA per drop, while liposome sprays usually contain 7.5 mg per spray.

Note: In this method of delivery, the hormone bypasses the liver, and a significant amount of DHEA is able to enter the general circulation. Be sure to adjust your dose for the different absorption rate that sublinguals have from capsules.

Creams

The assimilation and absorption rate is between 50 and 85 percent. Absorption is also directly into the bloodstream, again avoiding the liver. The absorption rate depends on the quality of the cream, what carriers are present, where on the body the cream is applied (areas where skin is thinner or areas of fatty tissue), the cleanliness of the skin, and the humidity.

Supplementing With DHEA

DHEA is most often taken in the form of capsules, which come in 5 mg, 10 mg, 25 mg, and 50 mg dosages. Once absorbed, the DHEA travels to the liver, where much of it is converted into androgens and estrogen. Because of this, not all the DHEA ingested enters the general circulation. Micronized DHEA (the hormone broken into tiny particles) is more efficiently absorbed by the body because the small size of the particles allows them to enter first the lymphatic system and then the general circulation, initially bypassing the liver. Since DHEA is a fat-soluble hormone, it is better absorbed when taken with food. DHEA taken orally is quickly absorbed, and blood levels rise within one hour.

However, much still needs to be learned about optimal dosage, timing, and how the hormone is best administered. There is a question of whether it is appropriate to raise DHEA to youthful levels or simply to a level that is adequate, given a person's age. Clinical trials are under way; in the meantime, clinicians who regularly prescribe DHEA generally agree on a certain range of starting dosages and recommend a gradual increase if needed.

In my experience, I have found that DHEA supplementation may be most beneficial for women after menopause. Beginning dosages should range from 5-15 mg a day, then be increased by 5-10 mg a day, as needed. DHEA dosages in women should not exceed 25 mg per day.

Conversely, there is no reason for women who have not reached menopause or perimenopause to consider taking DHEA replacement therapy. Women with normal menstrual cycles have no need for supplementing with DHEA since their bodies are making sufficient amounts of this hormone. On occasion, I have younger female patients who do so, and I strongly advise against it.

Some physicians recommend taking DHEA in the morning to reflect the body's own production of the hormone by the adrenal glands. Taken later in the day, DHEA can have a stimulating effect and sometimes causes insomnia; however, for a person suffering from a condition such as chronic-fatigue syndrome, this energizing effect could be of benefit.

Note: Before beginning supplementation of DHEA, women should have a mammogram and Pap smear test done to avoid the risk of stimulating a pre-existing cancer of the reproductive tract, since DHEA will increase the levels of the major sex hormones.

If you elect to use DHEA without a physician's guidance, buy the lowest-dose products available in your health food store or pharmacy, begin to use it cautiously, and do not go above 25 mg on your own. Let your physician recommend dosages at higher levels, and be sure to carefully monitor the effects on your body.

A Caution on Taking DHEA

Before starting DHEA supplementation, it is imperative to measure the amount of DHEA in the blood, and during the course of treatment, DHEA levels should continue to be monitored as regularly as every month. In fact, I strongly recommend that any individual considering taking DHEA consult an informed health care professional before starting a regimen. Taking more than 50 mg of DHEA definitely requires supervision.

Side Effects

DHEA is generally considered safe when taken in recommended dosages of 25 mg or less. While some sensitive people may experience side effects with dosages as low as 5 mg, side effects usually occur only when DHEA is taken in much higher amounts. Anyone taking over 50 mg a day of DHEA should be under a physician's supervision. Elevated doses of DHEA can actually prevent the adrenal glands from making the quantity of DHEA they normally produce.

As DHEA is a precursor hormone, which side effects occur in women depends on whether DHEA is being converted to male or female sex hormones. This varies from woman to woman depending on her genetic predisposition. Side effects of DHEA supplementation can include emotional symptoms such as irritability and depression, or physical ones like headaches, menstrual irregularity, and fatigue. DHEA may also have a slight masculinizing effect, especially in older women, who may develop mild acne and, even more rarely, facial hair.

There may also be long-term side effects from using high doses of DHEA. If a person has a family history of certain cancers that are hormone dependent, such as prostate cancer in men and cancers of the ovary, uterus, and breast in women, the supplementation of DHEA may increase the risk of developing these types of cancer. DHEA may also affect reproduction; therefore, taking the hormone is not recommended for women who are pregnant or breast-feeding.

Physicians who prescribe hormones suggest that DHEA be taken in the morning, as the body appears to have its highest concentrations at that time. If you are taking any prescription or over-the-counter drugs, you should check with your physician for any possible negative interactions or dosage changes.

Recent reports indicate that some individuals who have taken dosages of between 25 and 50 mg for only three to four weeks have experienced irregularities in heart rhythm. This information reinforces the advice that, if you are self-medicating, you should start at very low doses and only attempt higher doses under the supervision of a medical doctor who specializes in hormone therapy.

By keeping your DHEA levels balanced, you not only improve the production of other important sex hormones, but you improve your overall health and well-being. By simply following the program I've outlined for you in these two chapters, you can maintain proper DHEA production for years to come.

1. Maintain healthy DHEA production at the central nervous system level with 5-HTP, tyrosine, and other supportive nutrients.
2. Support DHEA production in the adrenals and ovaries with glandulars, beta-carotene, vitamin C, vitamin B5, zinc, and magnesium.
3. Support adrenal health with herbs such as Rhodiola rosea, panax ginseng, Siberian ginseng, licorice root, and PABA.
4. Use biochemically identical natural DHEA.

Summary

I've discussed the myriad of ways you can support your own production of DHEA with a variety of neurotransmitters, glandulars, herbs, and important vitamins and minerals, all of which work to create healthy hormone levels and function. You have also learned how biochemically identical DHEA can give you that extra "zest" you may need to get back on track. I hope that you enjoy the many benefits that having healthy levels of DHEA can provide!

About Susan Richards, M.D.

Dr. Susan Richards is one of the foremost authorities in the fields of family medicine and alternative medicine. Dr. Richards has successfully treated many thousands of patients emphasizing alternative health and integrative medicine in her clinical practice. Her mission is to provide her patients with safe and effective alternative therapies to greatly enhance their health and well-being.

A graduate of Northwestern University Feinberg School of Medicine, she has served on the clinical faculty of Stanford University School of Medicine and taught in their Division of Family and Community Medicine.

Her Facebook page, Dr. Susan's Healthy Living, has over one million followers. She is also an ordained minister and her ministry receives over a million prayer requests for healing each year.

NOTES

NOTES

NOTES

NOTES

Made in the USA
San Bernardino, CA
14 August 2018